To Paige,
Happy reading to you!
With love,
Gayle Childress Greene
2021

BECAUSE YOU ARE MINE

by Gayle Childress Greene

Illustrated by
Tiffany Tallent

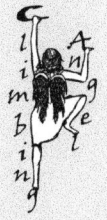

Because You Are Mine
by Gayle Childress Greene

Illustrated by Tiffany Tallent

Text & illustration copyright © 2021 Gayle Childress Greene

CAUTION: All rights reserved. No part of this publication may be reproduced, stored in a retrieval system, or transmitted in any form or by any means electronic, mechanical, photocopy, recording, or other, except for brief quotations in written reviews, without the prior written permission of the publisher.

Published in 2021 by:
Climbing Angel Publishing
PO Box 32381, Knoxville, Tennessee 37930
www.ClimbingAngel.com

First Edition May 2021
Printed in the United States of America

Cover layout by Jon Bonjour
Interior by Climbing Angel Publishing

ISBN: 978-1-63732-617-6

For my grandchildren...

Tyler
Ryan
Sienna
Aria

...because they are mine.

——————

Because You Are Mine

There could be lots of children

in a room...

...but I could find you.

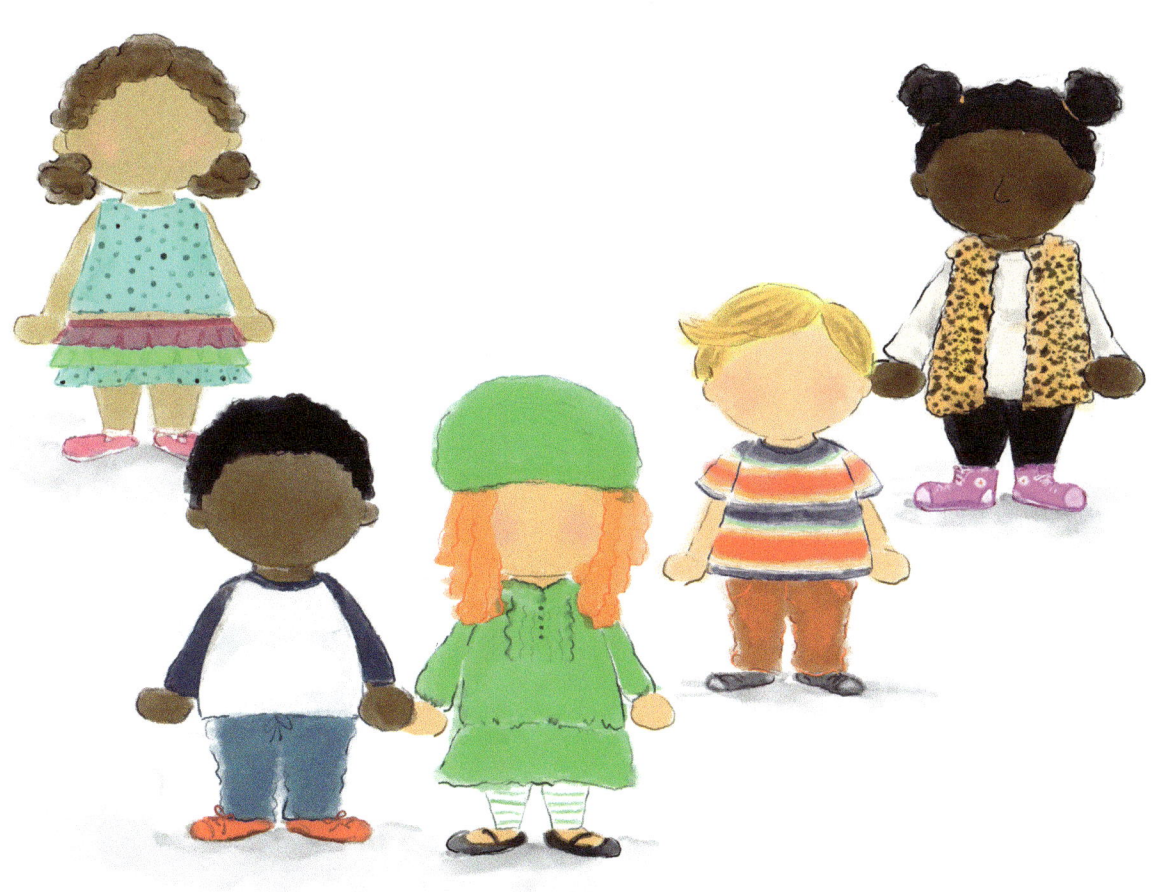

I would know you by your

nose!

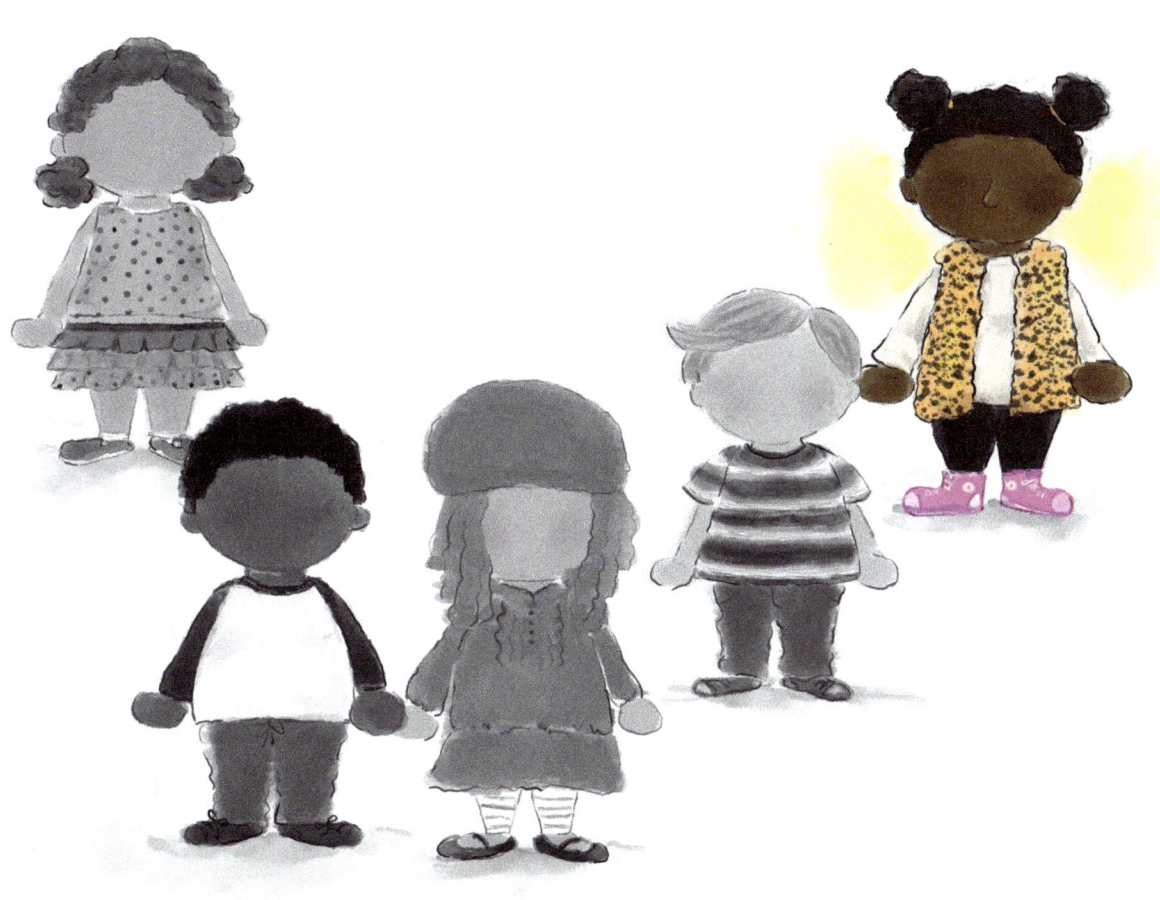

There could be lots and lots

of children in a room...

...but I could find you.

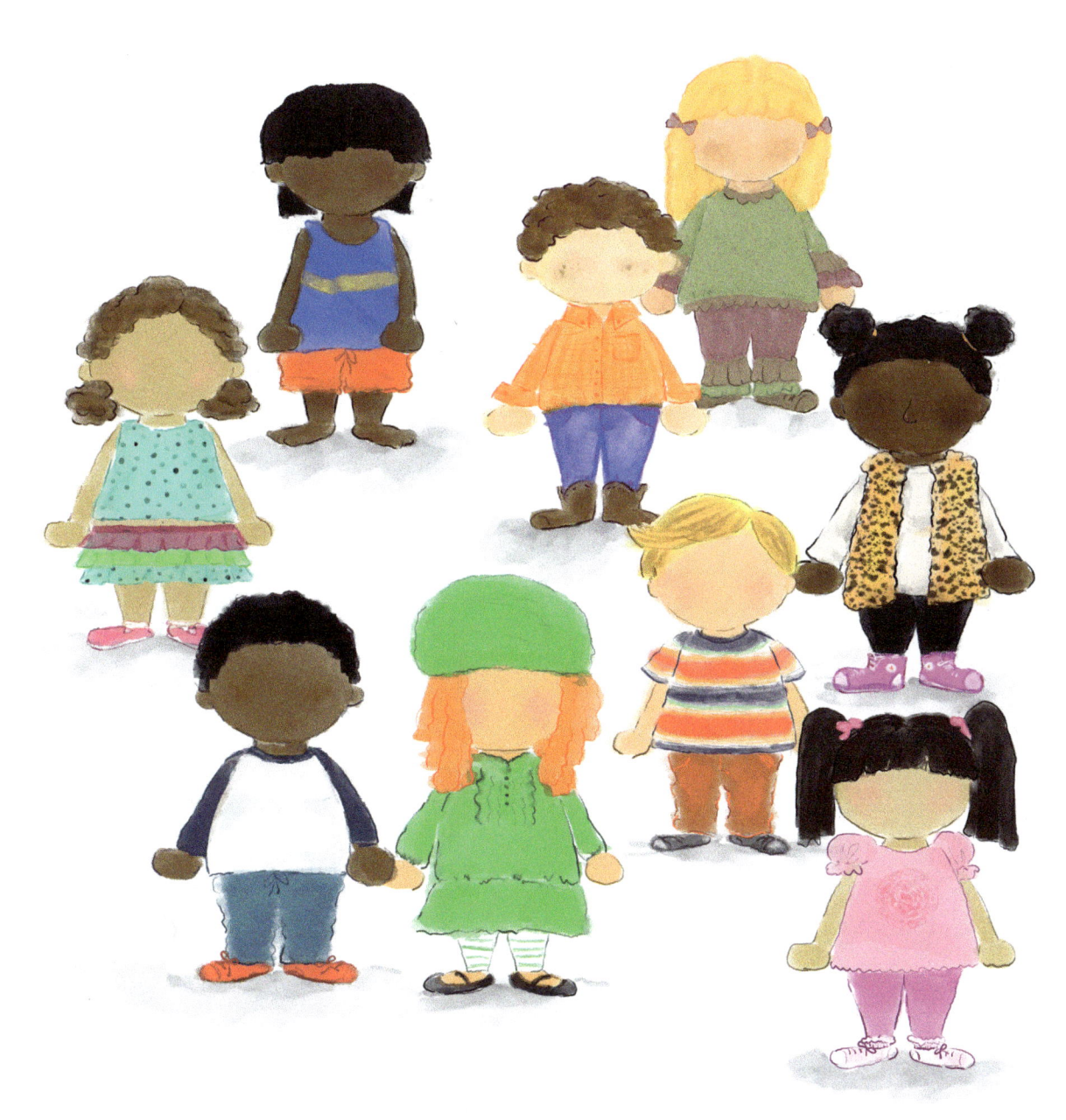

I would know you by your

toes!

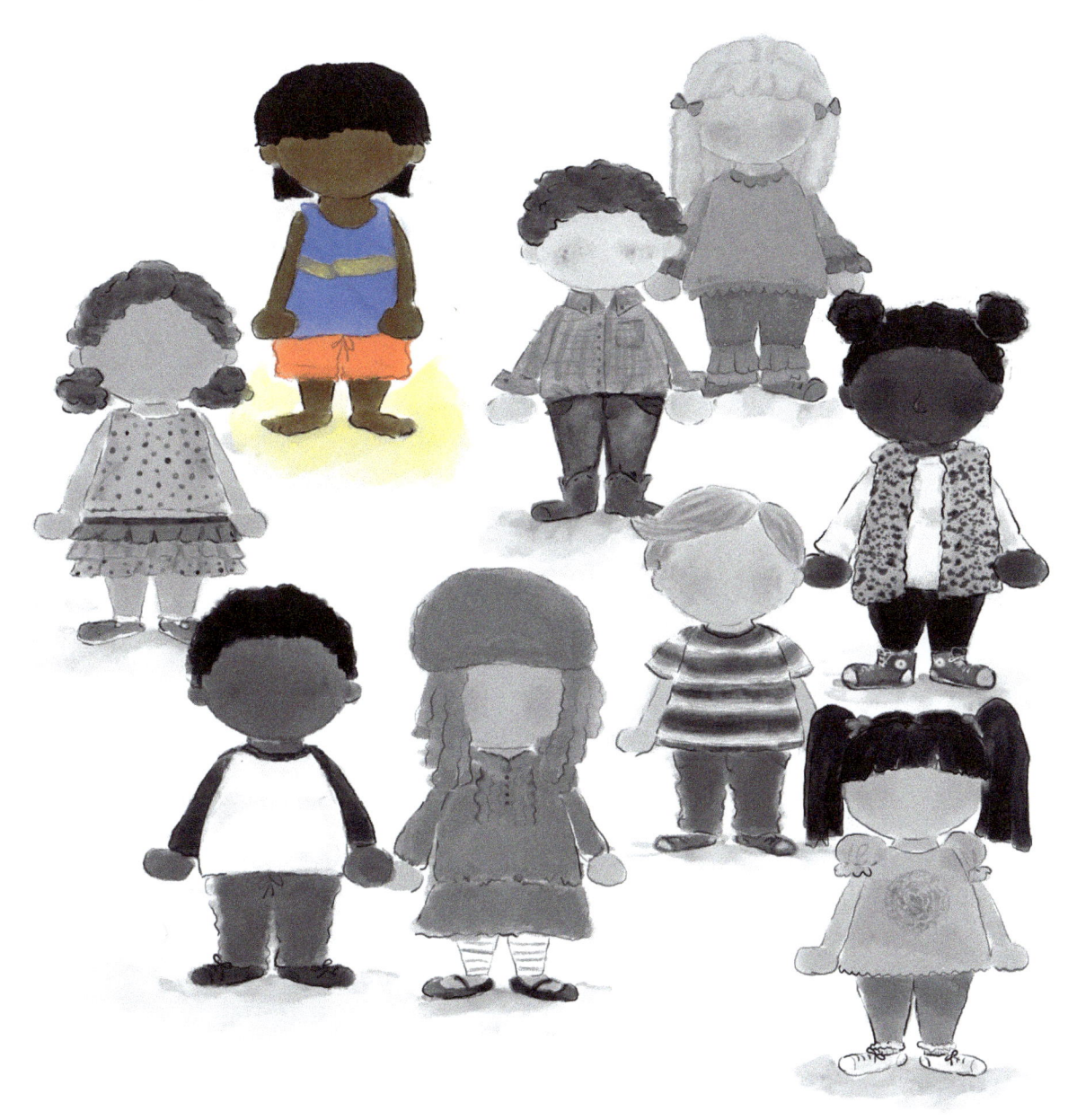

There could be lots
and lots
and lots of children
in a room...

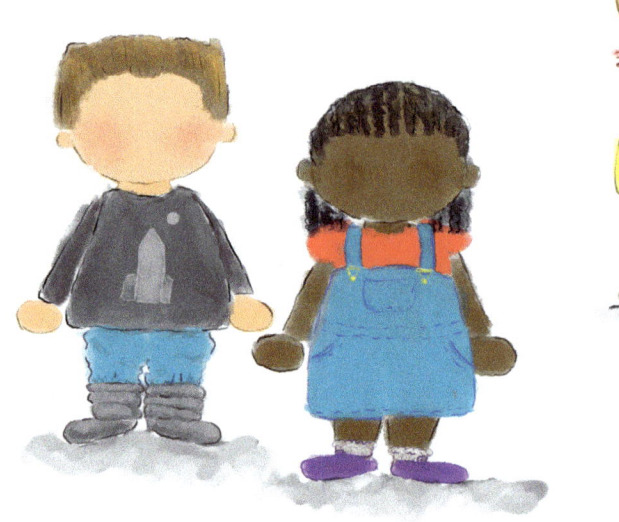

...but I could find you.

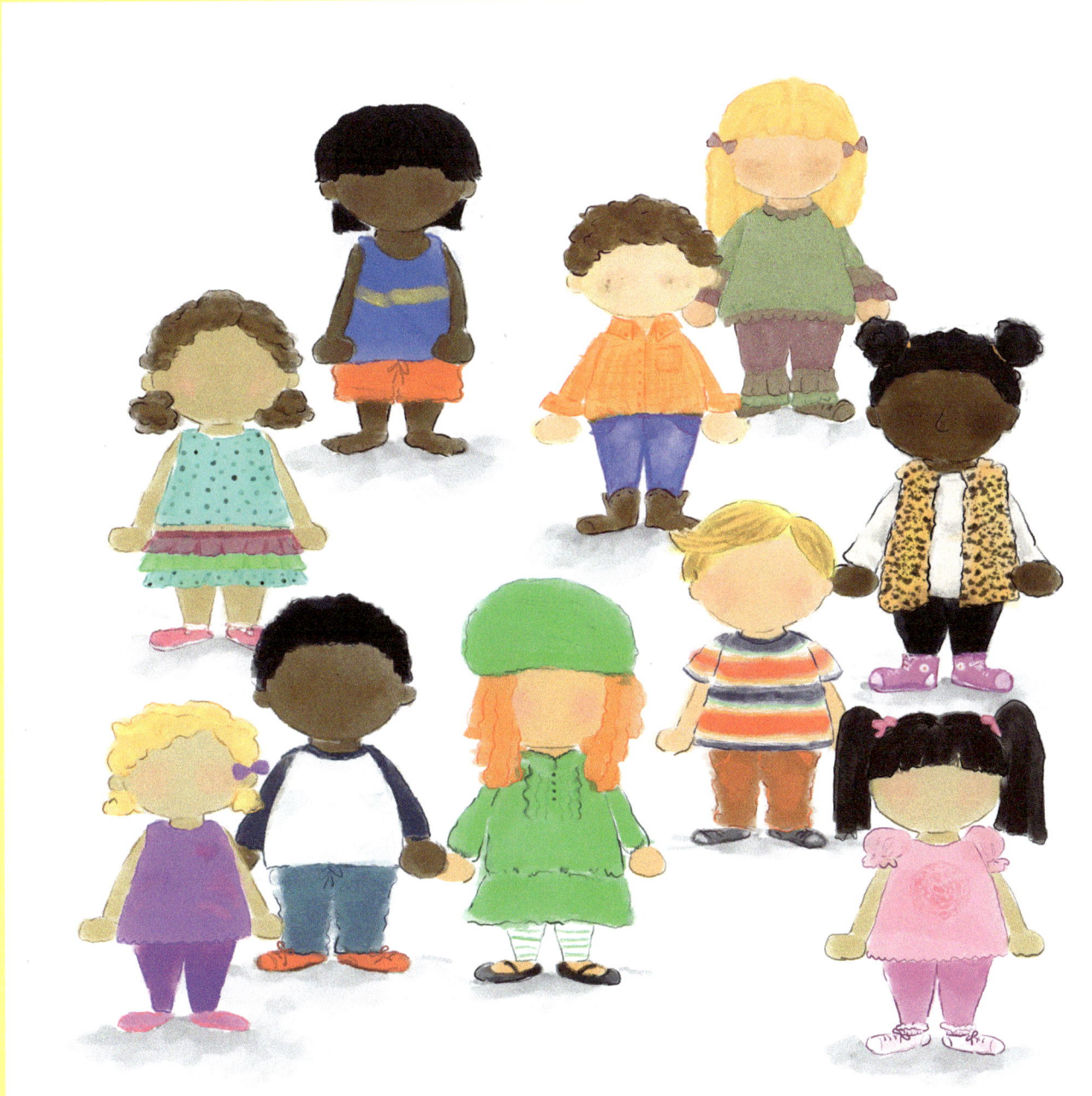

I would know you by your
chin!

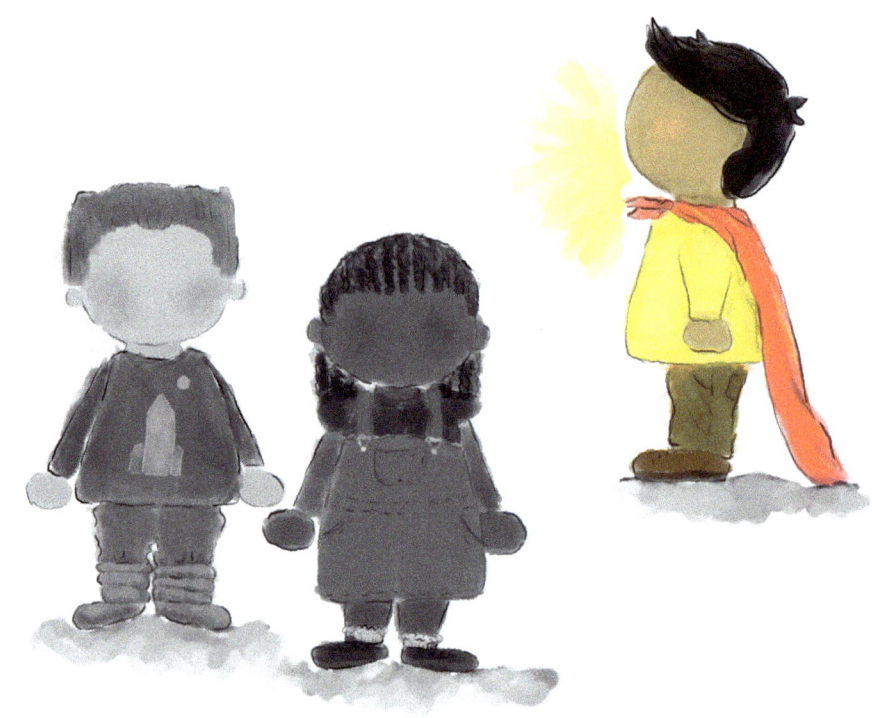

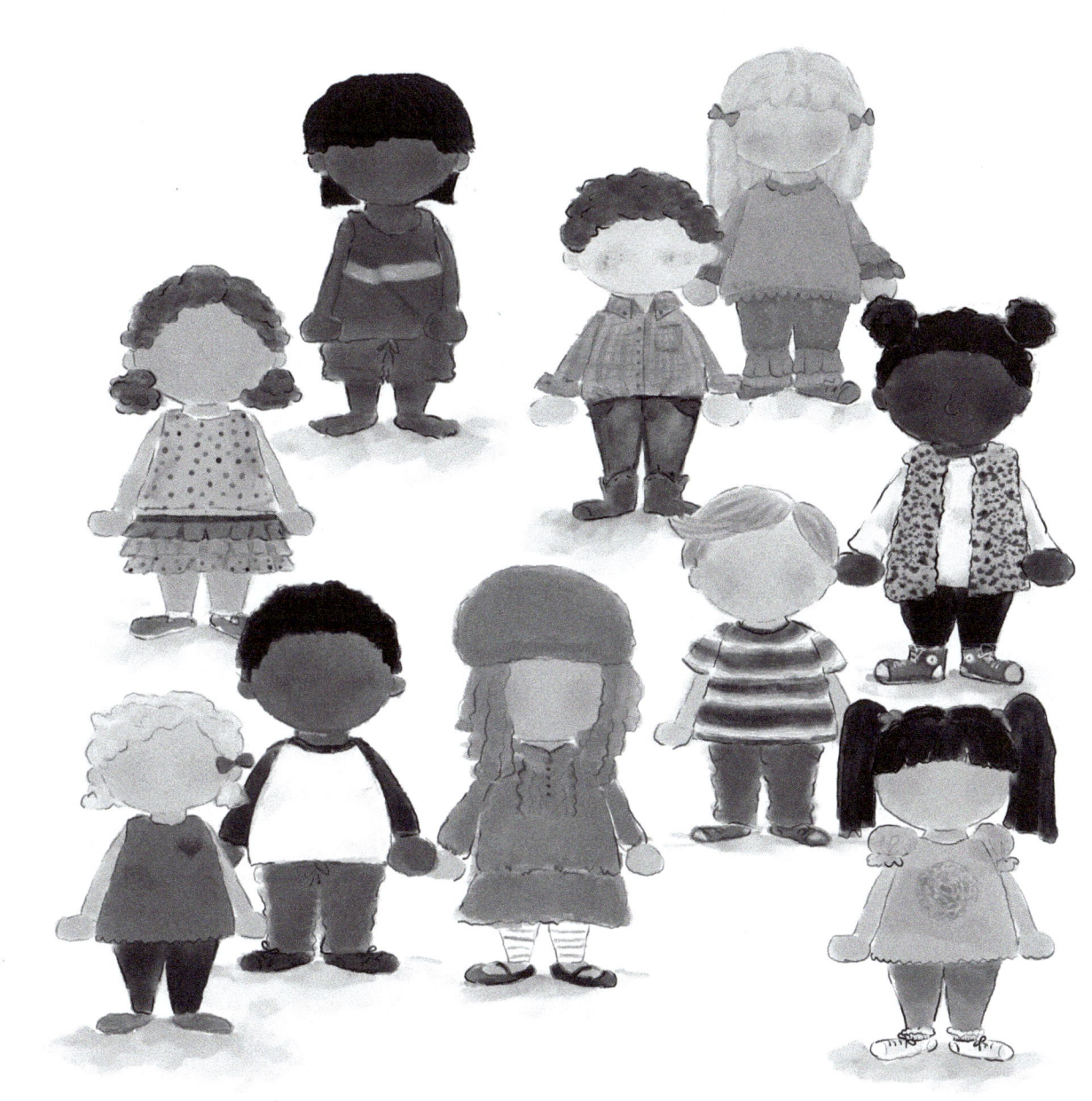

There could be LOTS and LOTS and LOTS and LOTS of children in a room...

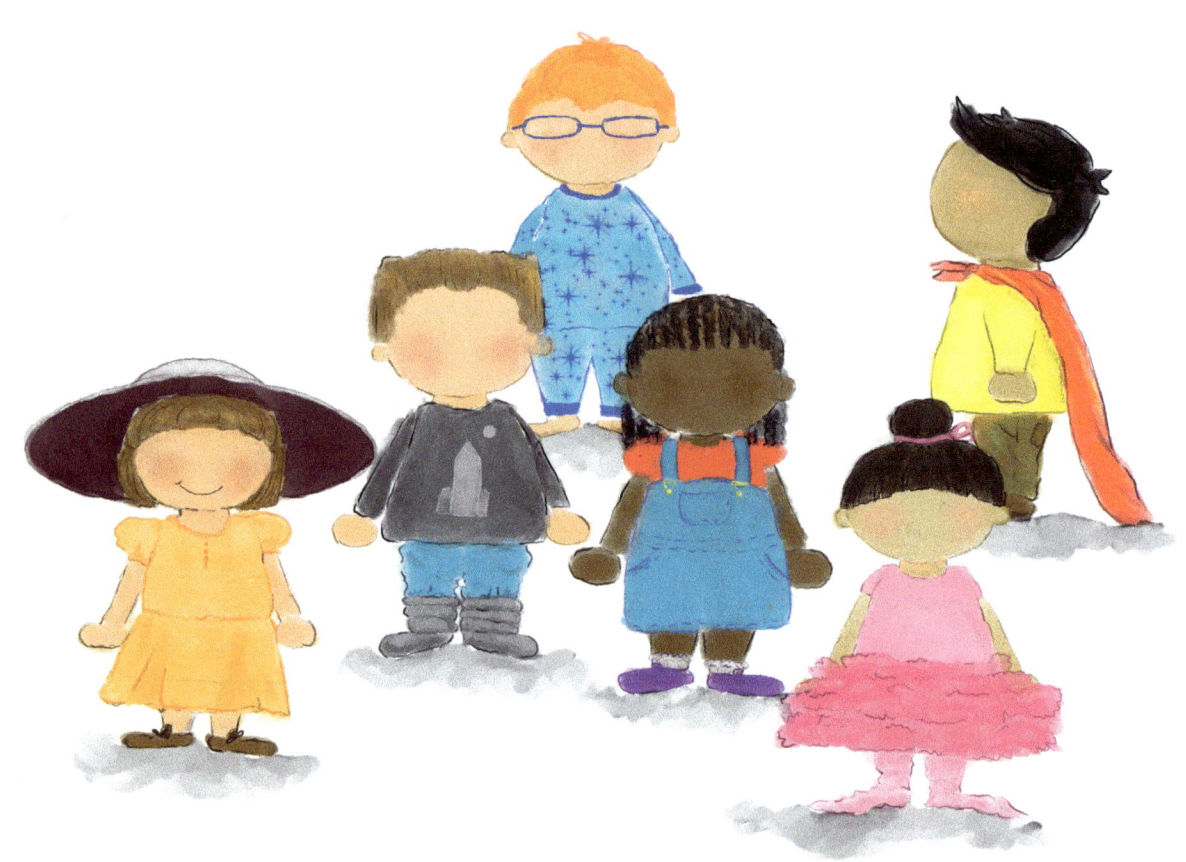

...but I could find you.

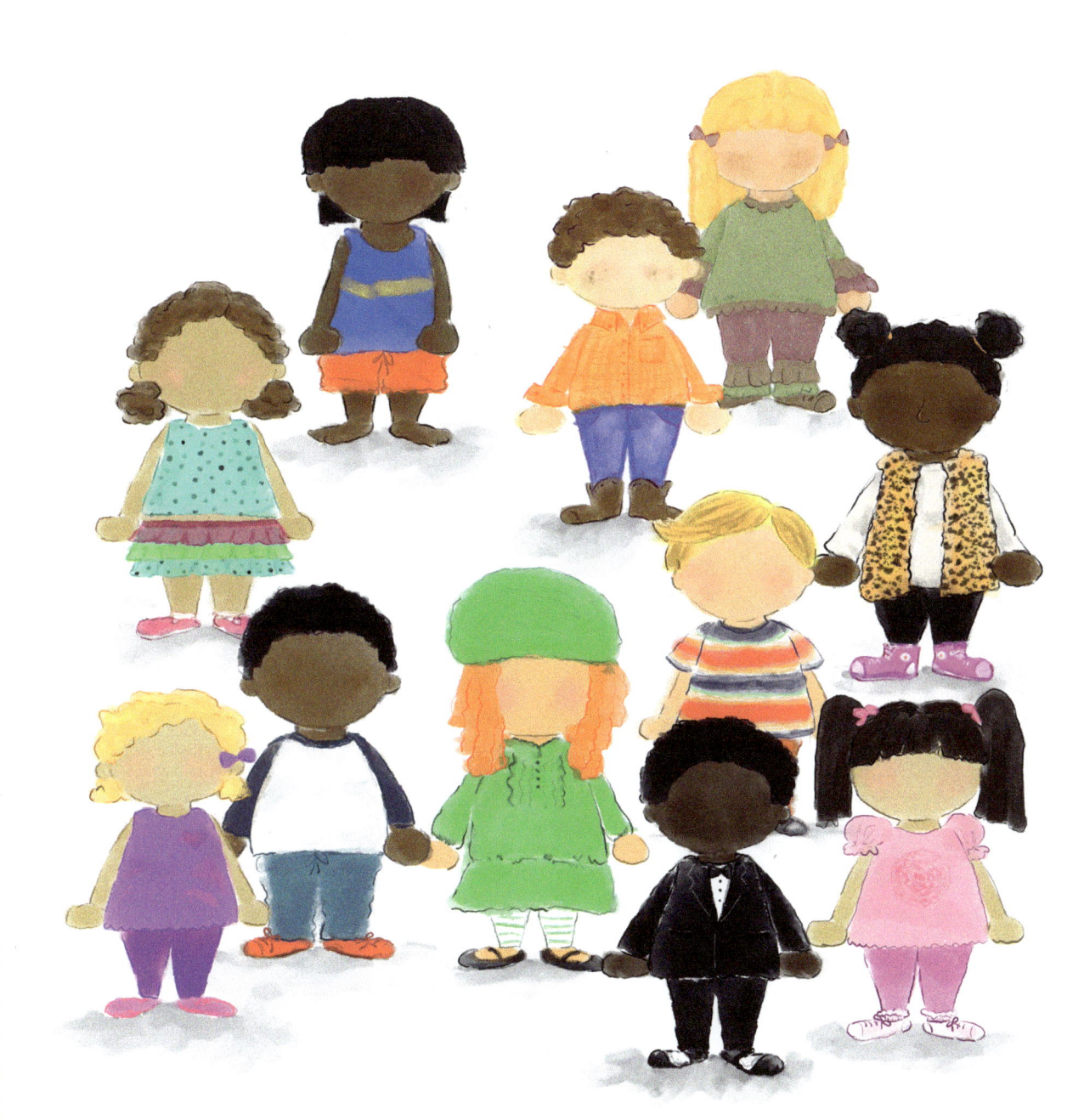

I would know you by your
grin!

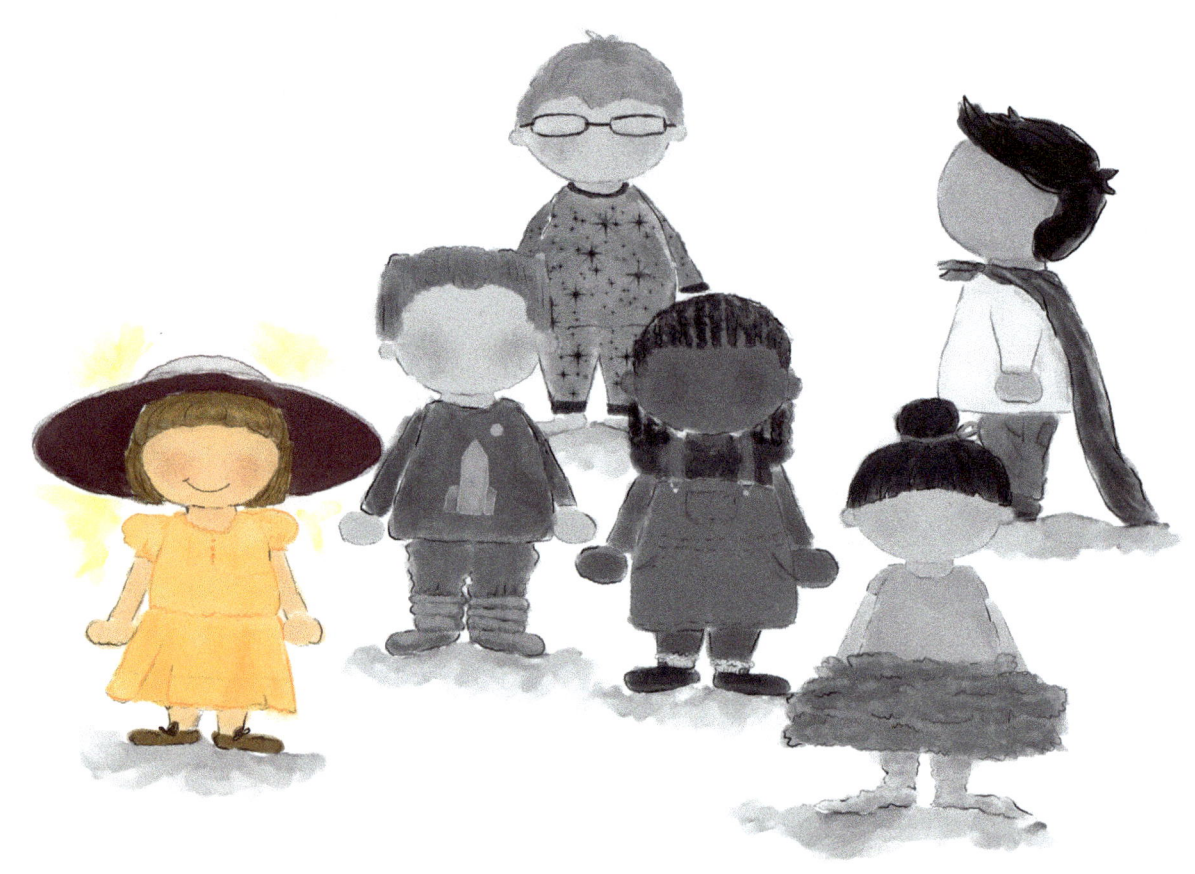

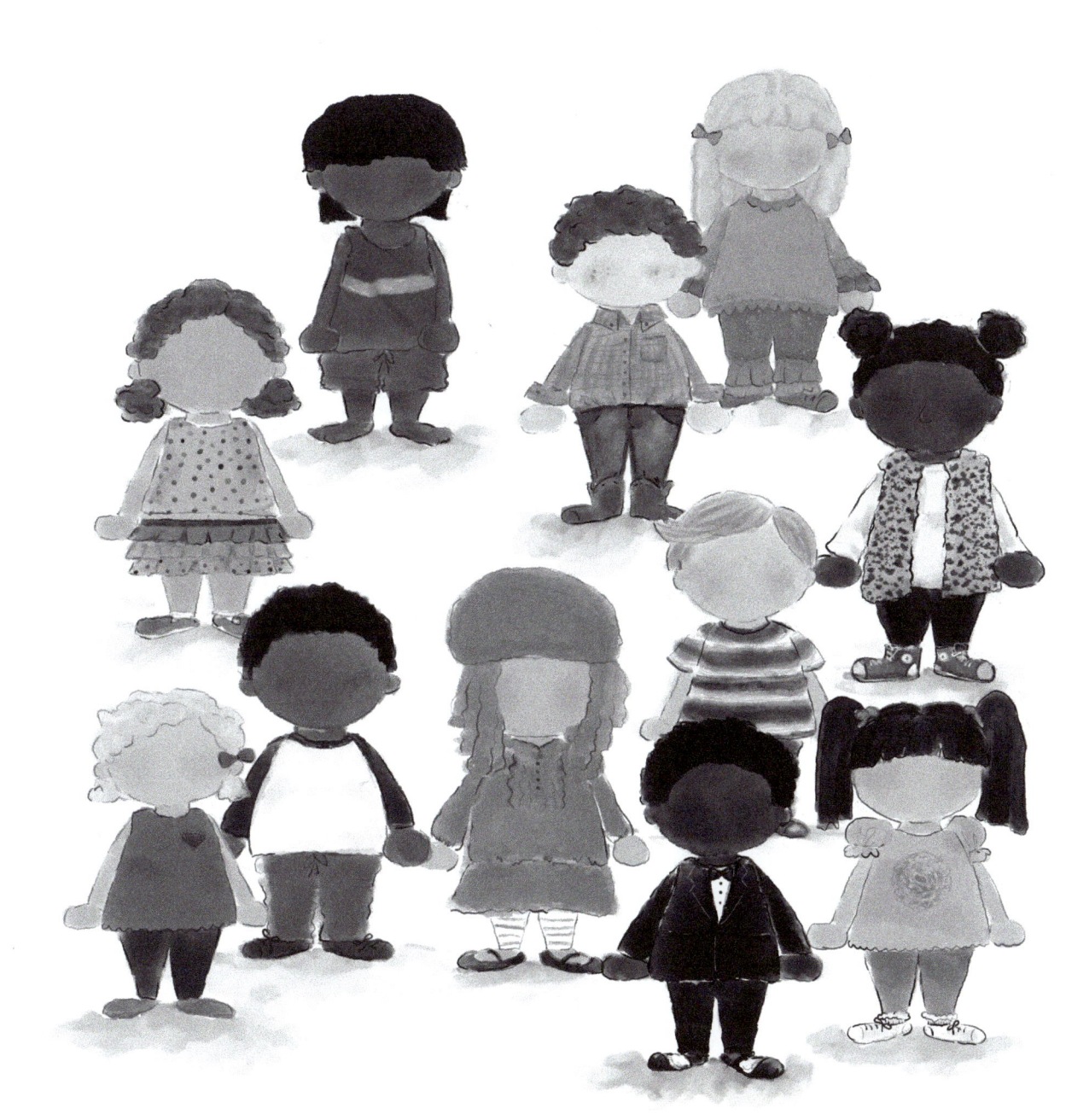

There could be LOTS and LOTS and LOTS and LOTS and LOTS of children in a room...

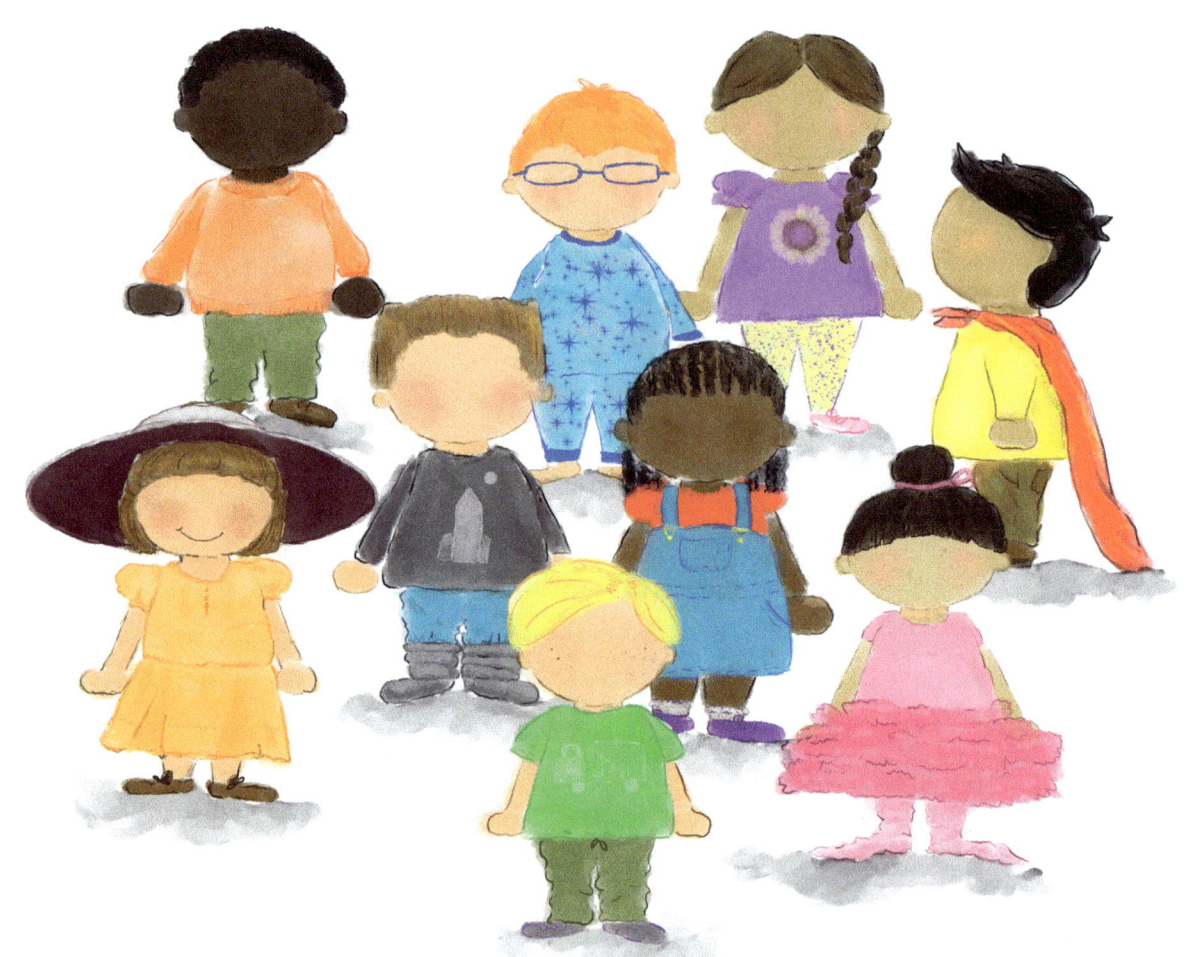

...but I could find you.

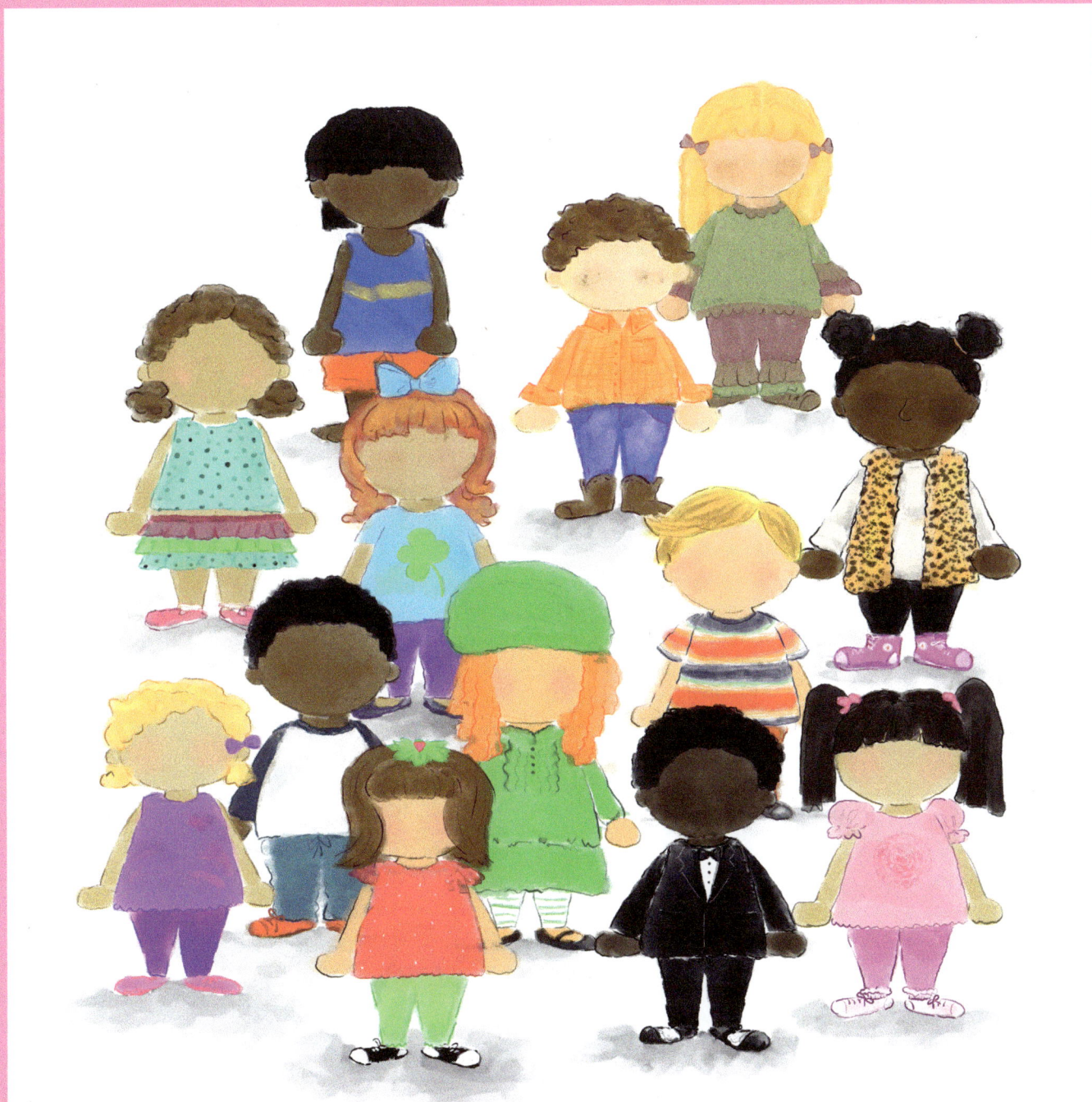

I would know you by your giggle...

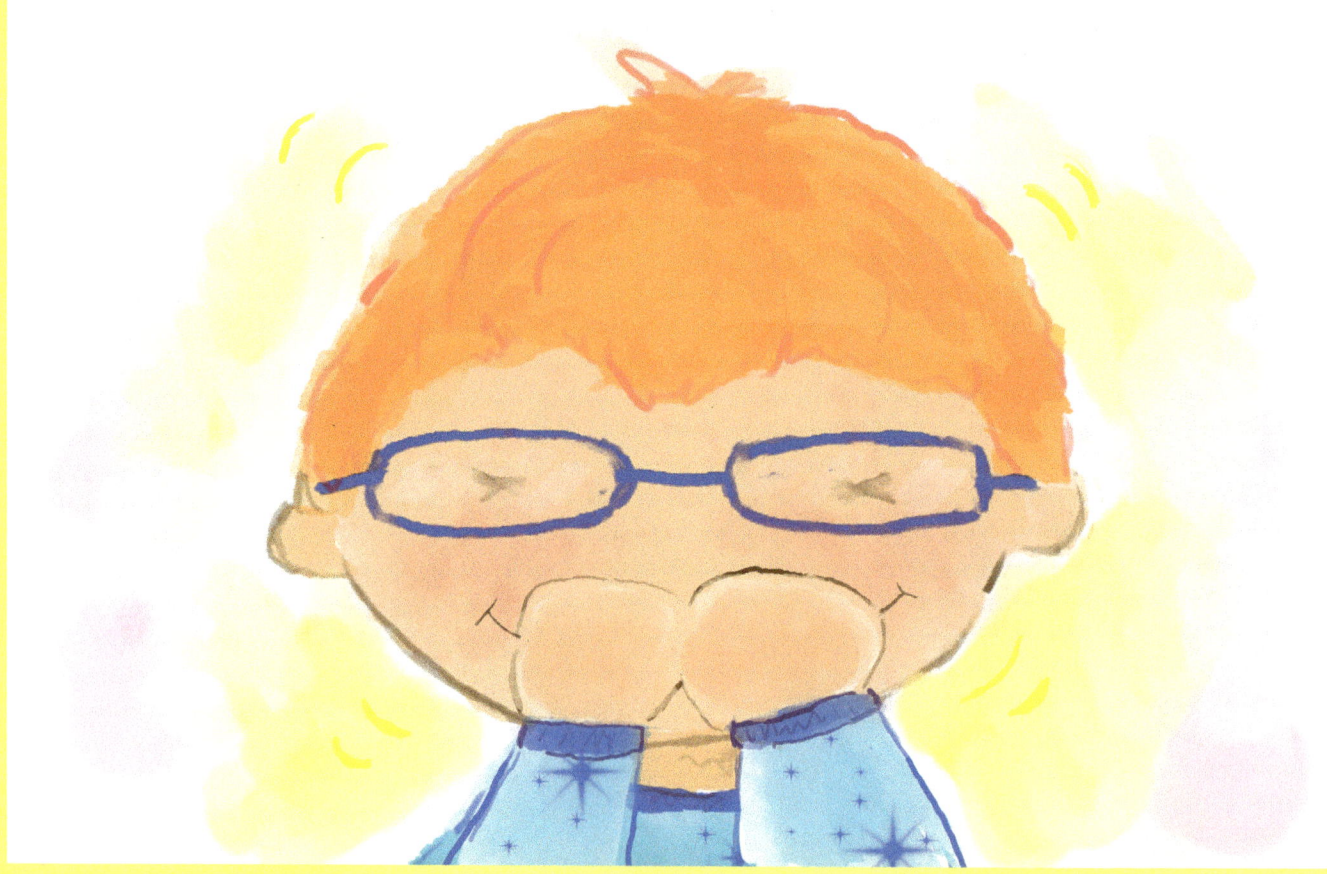

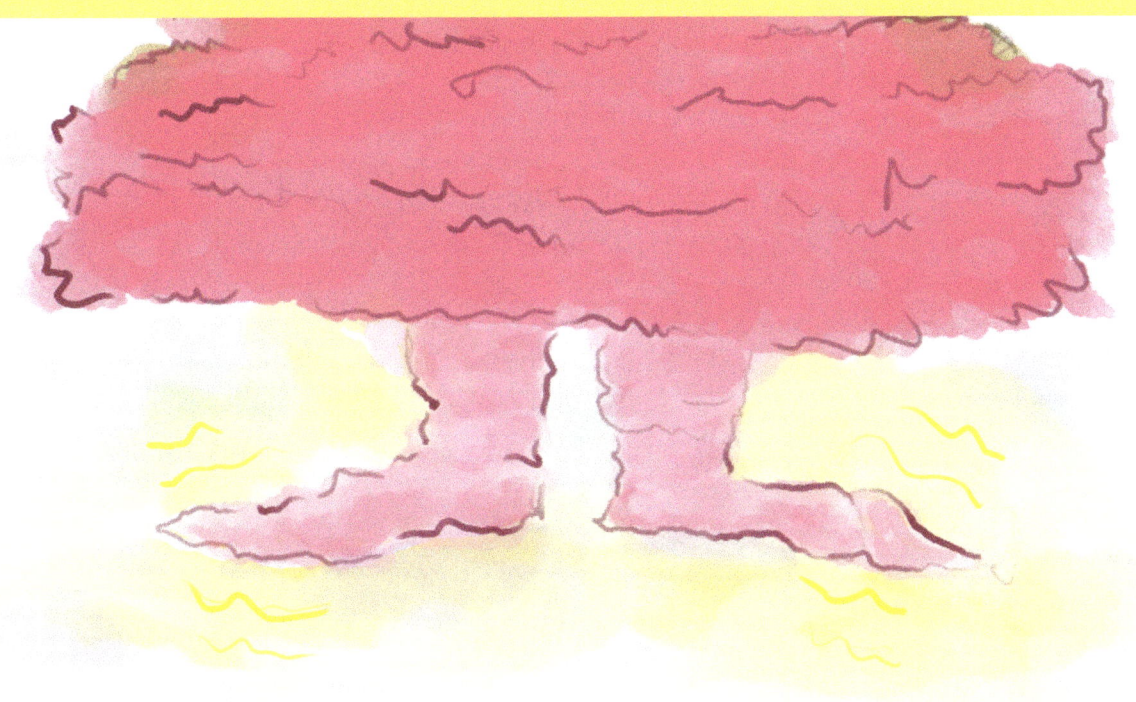

...and I would know you
by your wiggle!

I would know you in the
LIGHT...

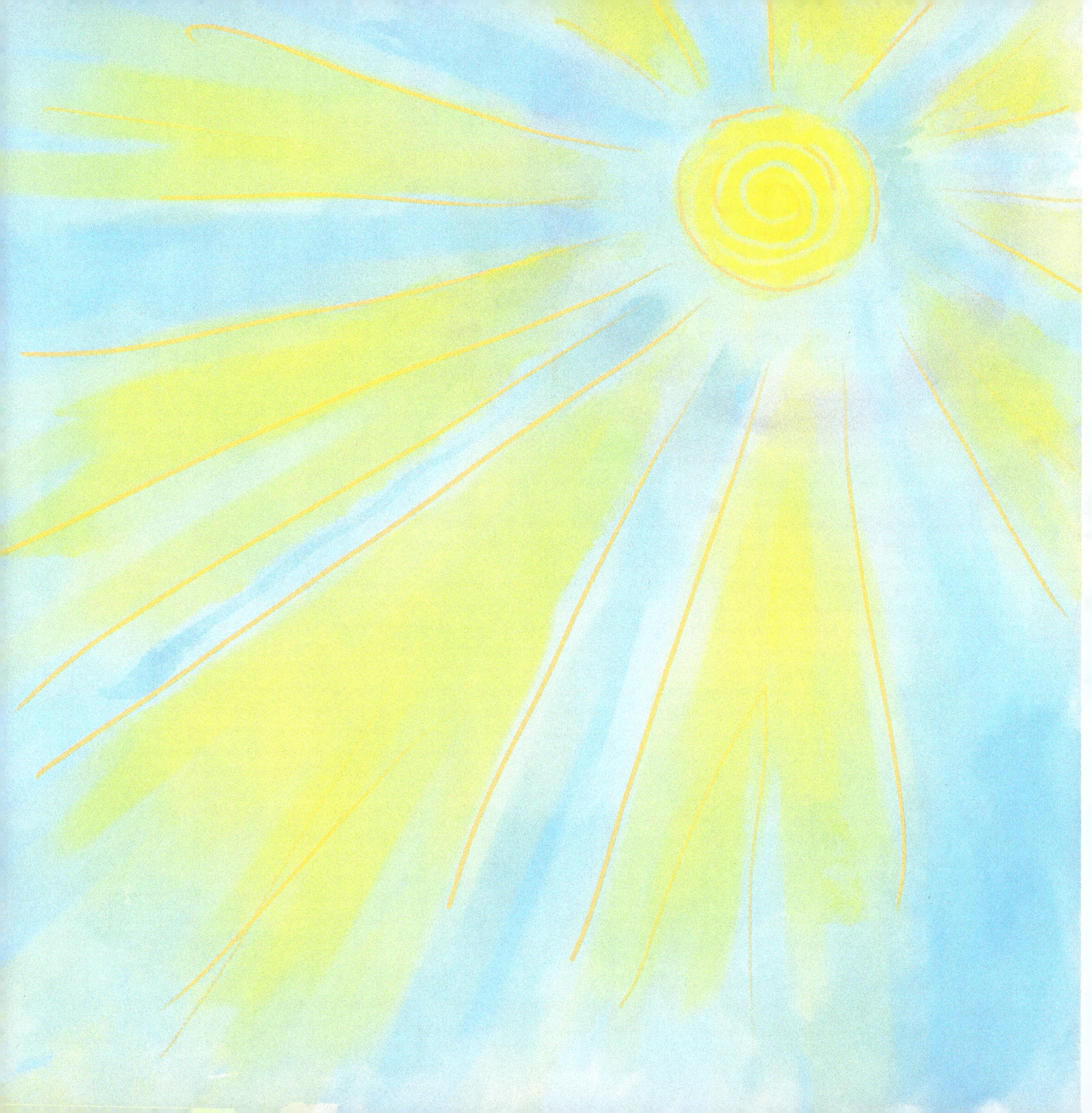

...and I would know you

in the NIGHT!

Even with my eyes closed

very, very TIGHT!

I would know you...

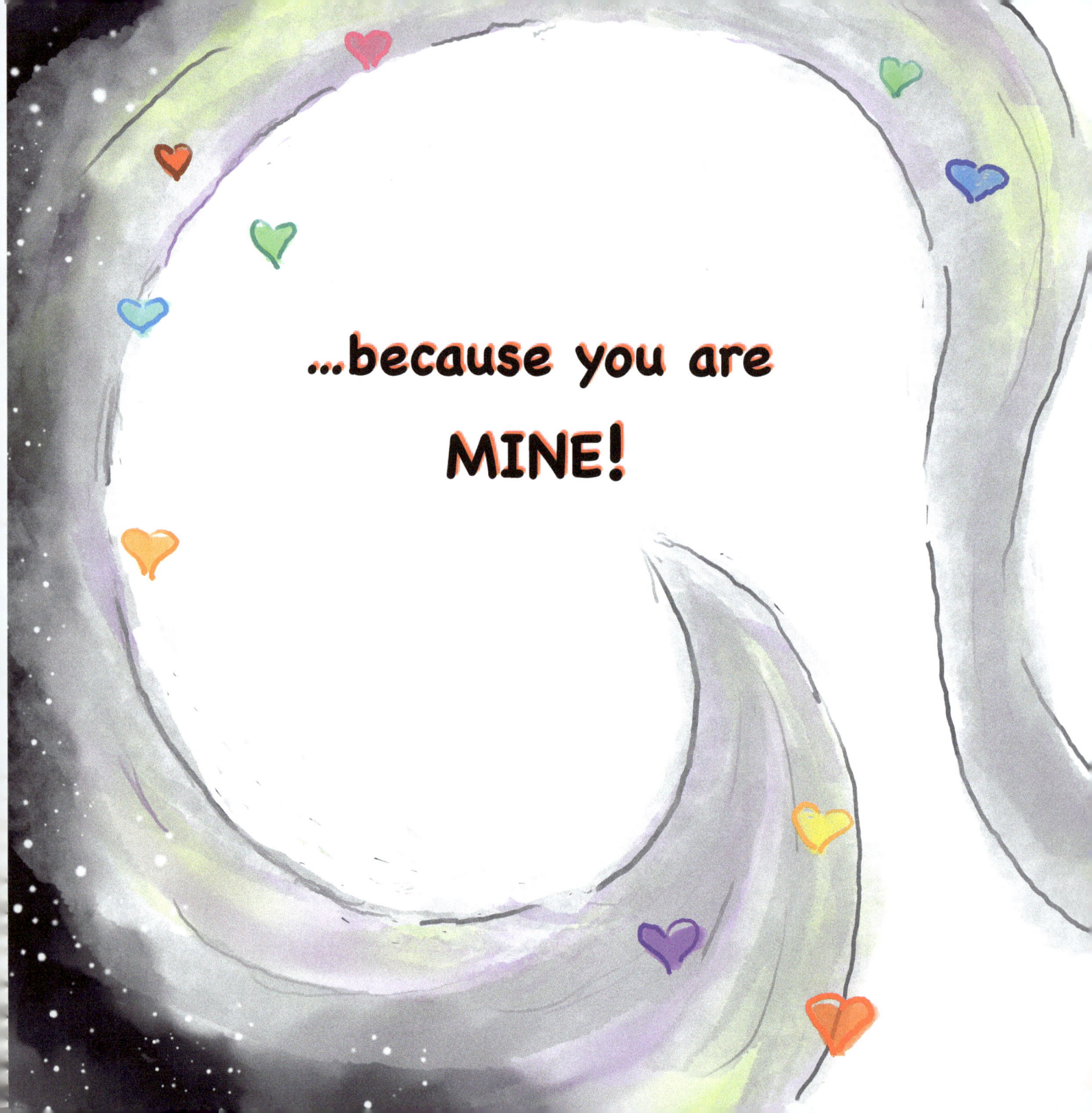

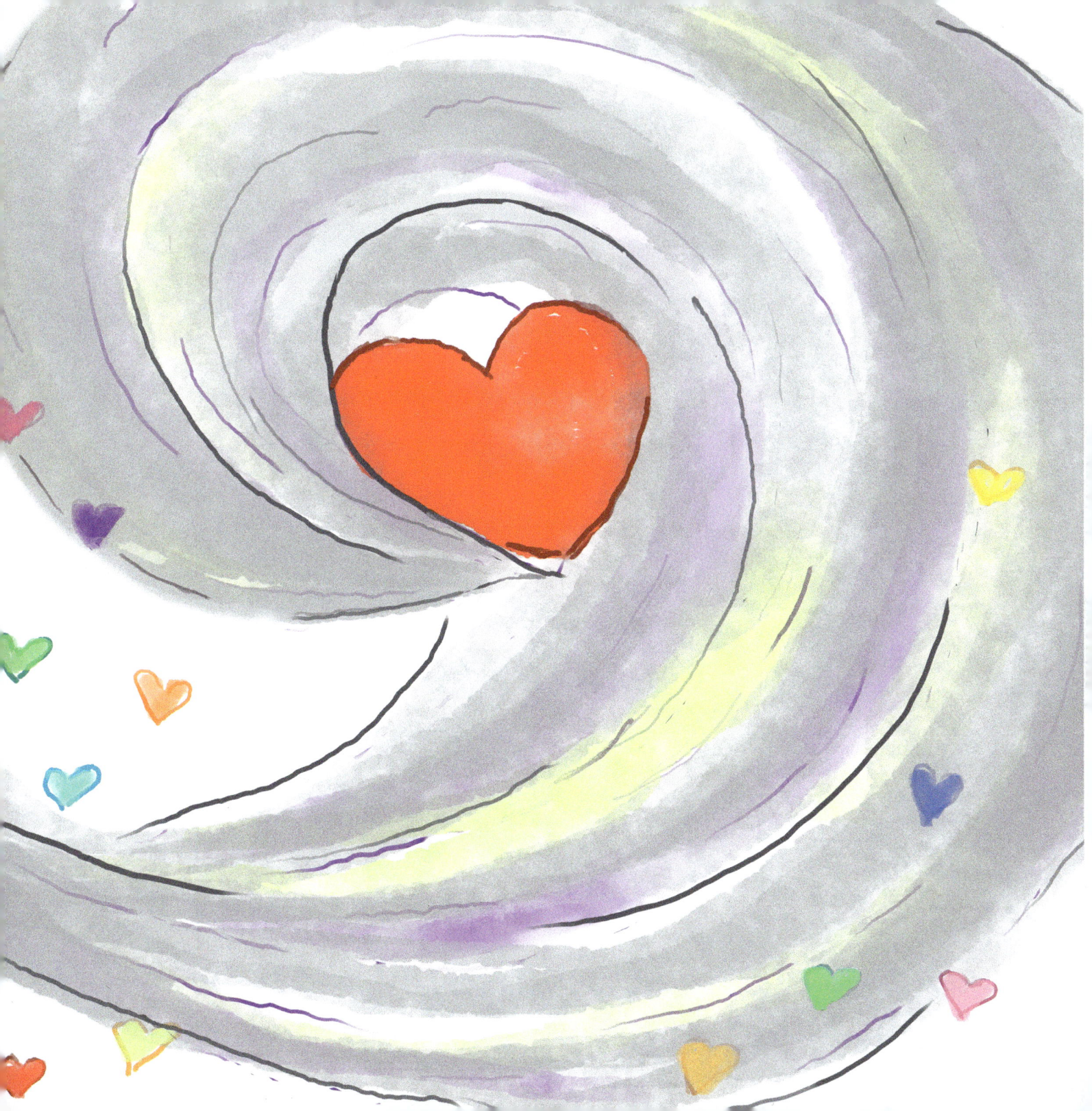

"For you formed my inward parts;
you knitted me together in my mother's womb.
I praise you, for I am fearfully and wonderfully made.
Wonderful are your works;
my soul knows it very well."

(Psalm 139:13-14, ESV)

The End

ABOUT CLIMBING ANGEL PUBLISHING

Climbing Angel Publishing exists for the purpose of sharing stories of hope and encouragement, aiding in the gathering together of community, and supporting the process of betterment. The following books are available at ClimbingAngel.com and major bookstores.

ADULT BOOKS: *(Romans 8:28-30)*

In His Image, Sam Polson (English, Romanian, & Mandarin)
By Faith, Sam Polson (English & Romanian)
My Birthday Gift to Jesus, Lisa Soland
Without Ceasing, Dr. Dennis Davidson
SonLight: Daily Light from the Pages of God's Word, Sam Polson
Corona Victus: Conquering the Virus of Fear, Sam Polson
Art Bushing: His Diary, Letters, & Photographs of WWII, Art Bushing
Art & Dotty: His Diary, Their Letters & Photographs of WWII, Art Bushing
Trimisul, Stan Johnson (Romanian)
Life Changing Prayer, Sam Polson

CHILDREN'S BOOKS: *(Philippians 4:8)*

The Christmas Tree Angel, Lisa Soland
The Unmade Moose, Lisa Soland
Thump, Lisa Soland
Somebunny To Love, Lisa Soland (English & Mandarin)
The Truth about God's Rainbow, Lisa Soland
God's Promises, Lisa Soland
The Boy & The Bagel Necklace, Lisa Soland
God's Hands and Feet, Lisa Soland
I Like To Be Quiet, Joni Caldwell
Wheels Off!, Karlie Saumier
Ella's Trip of a Lifetime, Melanie Ewbank
Because You Are Mine, Gayle Childress Greene

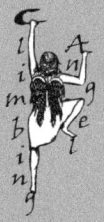

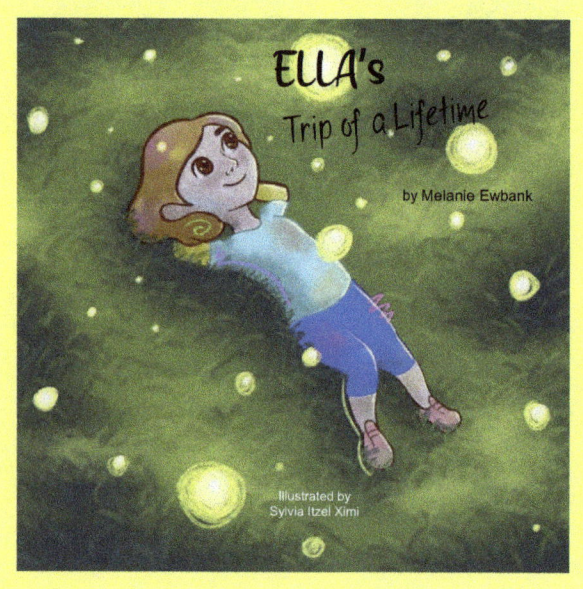

ELLA'S TRIP OF A LIFETIME
by Melanie Ewbank

ELLA IS A KID WHO NEEDS TO STAY ACTIVE. SHE GETS BORED EASILY. Her mom says, "Ella, you have a family of squirrels in your brain that seems to be impossible to manage." During a family vacation, Ella's impatience gets the best of her, and she tries to swim in the hotel pool by herself. Ella nearly drowns, then takes the trip of a lifetime to visit heaven. While there, she learns a lesson she will never forget!

WHEELS OFF!
by Karlie Saumier

Wheels Off! is Hazel and Henry's first of many adventures together. Henry is Hazel's little brother, who sometimes wishes he wasn't so little. While playing at the local playground, a group of bullies pick on Henry, but his sister is there to help him discover that "Heaven on Earth" is not that far away.

"A terrific Christ-inspired story of forgiveness, family, and friendship."
– Lisa Soland, author

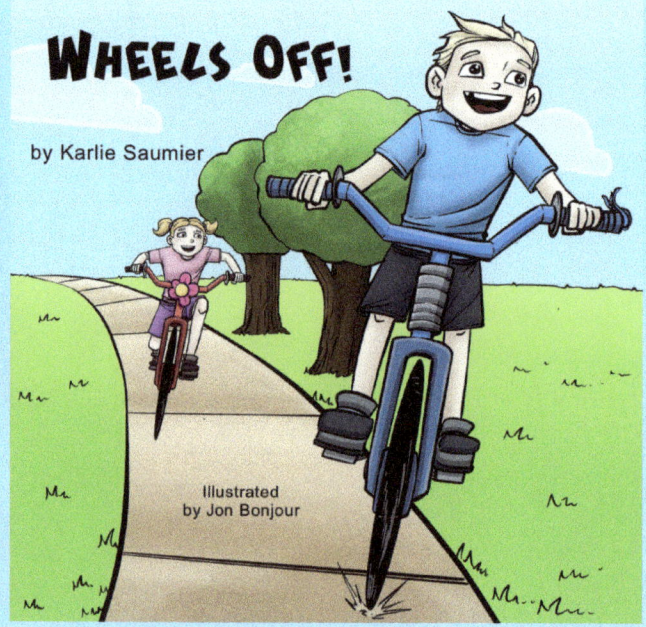

I LIKE TO BE QUIET
by Joni Caldwell

This book is written to honor *the quiet child*, the child that likes to observe, the child that enjoys a little alone time to think. Like me, I know you are amazed as you watch your quiet child. I hope this book will serve as the backdrop for you to snuggle into each other for a while. Let's make sure they know how interesting they are and how very proud we are of them, *just the way they are.*

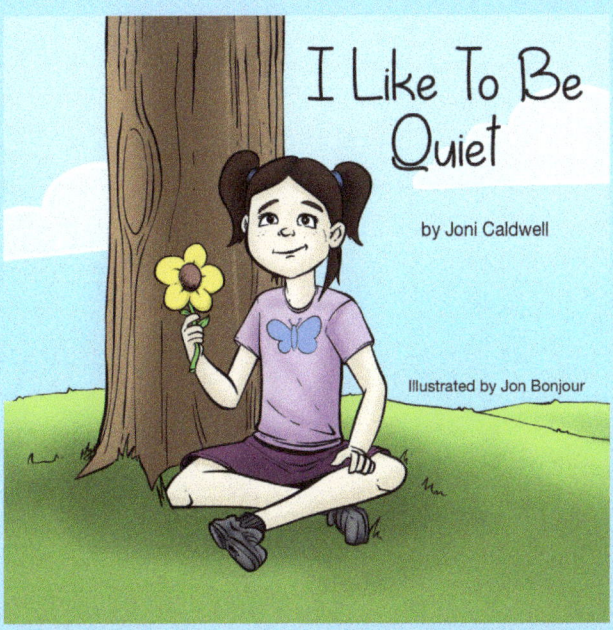

THE BOY & THE BAGEL NECKLACE
by Lisa Soland

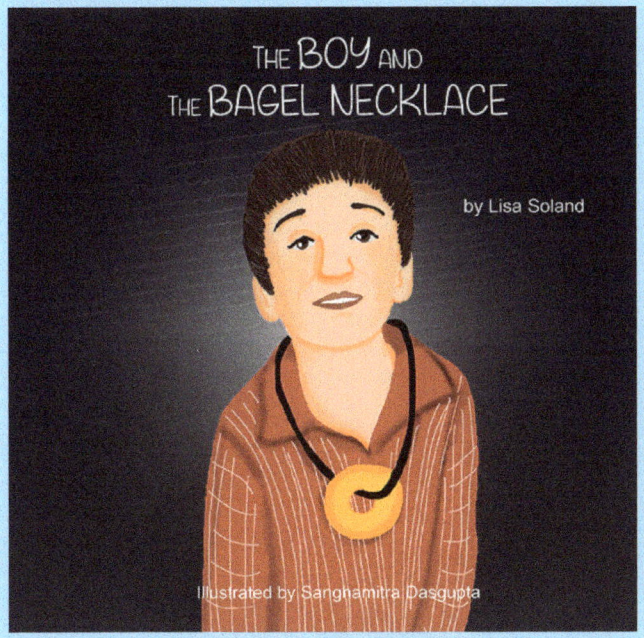

In *The Boy and the Bagel Necklace*, Andrew, a resident of a Romanian orphanage, tells us the story of when Jesus visited him in a dream. Jesus tells Andrew not to worry, that everything is going to be all right. Soon after, the leadership in Romania changes and little Andrew is adopted and brought to America where he learns that Jesus Christ is more than just a nice man who visits desperate children in their dreams. When little Andrew learns just how much God loves him, his life is radically changed.

CPSIA information can be obtained
at www.ICGtesting.com
Printed in the USA
LVHW072108200421
685063LV00001B/1